POWERFUL WEIGHT LOSS STRATEGIES

(www.mitchfitness.com)

DISCLAIMER AND TERMS OF USE AGREEMENT

This Book is a general educational health-related information product. As an express condition to reading to this eBook, you understand and agree to the following terms.

The Book content is not a substitute for direct, personal, professional medical care and diagnosis. None of the exercises mentioned in this Book should be performed nor the nutritional advice used without clearance from your physician or health care provider.

There may be risks associated with participating in activities or using products mentioned in this Book for people in poor health or with pre-existing physical or mental health conditions.

Because these risks exist, you will not use such advice or take part in such activities if you are in poor health or have an existing mental or physical condition.

If you choose to ignore these risks, you do so of your own free will and accord, knowingly and voluntarily assuming all risks associated with such activities.

If you do not agree with these terms and express conditions, do not read this Book. Your use of this Book, products, or services, and any participation in activities mentioned in this eBook, means that you are agreeing to be legally bound by these terms.

You agree to hold the Author of this book, the Author's owners, agents, affiliates, and employees harmless from any and all claims, demands, rights of action or causes of action, present or future,

First published as an ebook by Mitchell Okotie via kindle Direct Publishing in JUNE 20, 2012.

CONTENTS

About the Author

Mitchell Okotie *(personal training fitness expert).* **I have been in the fitness industry for over twenty years, and qualified with the London YMCA personal training award in 1998. I have been in the business with the main goal of helping people around the world learn the best way to lose weight effectively and how to build a better body and improve their health.**

My main goal in writing this book is to empower you, the reader, toward your personal fulfillment and happiness as regards losing weight and attaining a better body and health through the best formulas of "how-to." To you and to millions of people around the world who would like to lose weight, may this book be a light, and a guide for you to follow so that you can be the person that deep down you would really love to be.

The whole idea of writing this first book, and several other books over the past eight years that are soon to be published, is to bring to light the great negative effects of weight gain and what we can all do to overcome those weight gain issues.

The main reason why I have been so passionate about weight loss is that I have not been in any way exempt from putting on weight, especially as I reached the thirties mark. When I was eighteen years of age up until thirty, I could eat tons of food and not really put on weight because I was regularly exercising, but that all changed when I reached the age of thirty.

From then on for many years it was a constant struggle. I did put on weight FAST, 4 pounds, 8 pounds, and at times more. Whenever I put on weight, I did not feel good in any way. It affected my mood; it took away my true happiness; it de motivated me; it made me look less attractive; it made me feel really sluggish;

and at times I felt trapped – trapped because I could not break out of those eating and drinking habits that I really loved tremendously.

That was a time that I had to find and develop the most effective and powerful ways to overcome weight gain and lose weight FAST with immediate effect. I now knew the most powerful ways to do so, being able to lose up to 8 pounds within a week, and I started to be able to convey this great knowledge of how to lose weight FAST to thousands of clients who I have come across and helped over the years. Many of those who took my advice lost weight FAST whether they were in their twenties, thirties or forties.
The principles and understanding of losing weight FAST is going to work for you, if you are prepared to make it work. I really wish you all the best on your journey of losing weight and attaining a better body and improving your health.

INTRODUCTION

In this book, I am going to show you the most powerful ways for you to lose weight **FAST** around the areas of your body that you are not happy with. The most powerful weight loss strategies revealed are as follows:

1. Goal setting.
2. The right type of diet.
3. The right type of training program for fast weight loss.
4. The right use of techniques, visualization, and focus.
5. Your mindset.
6. Taking action.
7. Determination.
8. Consistency and commitment.
9. Discipline.
10. Patience.
11. Relaxation.
12. The achievement of your goals.

THE POWER OF GOAL SETTING

Over the course of many years, I have come across and helped thousands of people who have had the goal of wanting to lose weight FAST. Most people who need to lose weight know that the best way for them to do so is to be on a good diet plan and to exercise regularly.

When setting out to lose weight, it is very important for you to have clear and specific goals of the amount of weight that you would like to lose (toward your target weight) which could be for example 8 pounds, 14 pounds, 21 pounds or more. Once you have decided, you need to have a plan of ACTION. This will include the right type of diet to lose weight FAST in section 2 and also the right type of training program which is going to MAXIMIZE your weight loss process, in section 3.

The general guideline and goal for weight loss in the fitness industry is to lose 2 pounds each week in order for your weight loss process to become VERY SUCCESSFUL. In a four-week period, this is going to amount to 8 pounds of body FAT lost. This will be the minimum that you should achieve through my method and is definitely not the maximum that you can achieve.

If you are trying to lose weight but you are not losing at least 2 pounds of body FAT each week, it means that you are not achieving SUCCESS as far as your weight loss process is concerned. Weight gain for most people, me included, generally starts around the stomach area, and if it is not controlled it spreads to other parts of the body such as the face, the arms, the thighs, ankles, feet, and in short the whole body. This can lead to the following negatives in a person's life, for example:

a.   Insecurity.
b.   Very low self-esteem and confidence.
c.   Frustration.
d.   Stress.
e.   De motivation.
f.   Bad health.
g.   Unhappiness.
h.   Lack of energy.
i.   Depression.

If you are experiencing any of those negatives due to putting on weight, you should set an immediate goal RIGHT AWAY, to overcome any of those negatives, and to experience the total opposite, which is the following:

a.   Security.
b.   Higher self-esteem and confidence.
c.   No frustration.
d.   Joy.
e.   Motivation.
f.   Good health.
g.   Happiness.
h.   High levels of energy.
i.   Personal fulfillment.

And these positives can be attained by the ACHIEVEMENT of your weight loss goals, if you are going to IMPLEMENT the weight loss SUCCESS strategies that I talk about in the remaining part of this book.

THE RIGHT TYPE OF DIET

Food

These days, there is a huge amount of information about diets for losing weight. One thing is certain, most of the main diets talk about reducing food and carbohydrates greatly. Some talk about getting rid of meat, fish and chicken from your diet. Some diets say that you should not eat any fruits, or you should have a liquid only diet, while some advocate a fruit only diet.

The one that I want to talk about is the type of diet that is going to help you lose weight FAST, and at the same time leave you feeling light, full, and healthy. It will make you look younger, give you very good skin, and also greatly energize your body system. I want to show you several diet plans that you will be able to follow:

DIET PLAN ONE

Breakfast
2 slices of bread
2 eggs any style
1 glass of orange juice
1 glass of water

Lunch
Fish
1 baked potato
Salad
1 glass of water

Dinner
Chicken or steak
Vegetables
Salad
1 glass of water

DIET PLAN TWO

Breakfast
2 eggs any style
Oatmeal or porridge
1 glass of orange juice
1 glass of water

Lunch
Tuna
1 baked potato
Salad
1 glass of water

Dinner
Fish
Vegetables
Salad
1 glass of water

DIET PLAN THREE (WITHOUT MEAT)

Breakfast
2 eggs any style
A smoothie (blended fruits)
1 slice of wholegrain bread with a teaspoon of peanut butter
1 glass of water

Snack
Dried fruit or nuts, seeds

Lunch
1 slice of wholegrain bread
Vegetables
Salad
1 glass water

Dinner
Lentil soup

DIET PLAN FOUR:
STRICTER FOR FASTER WEIGHT LOSS

Breakfast
3 eggs
1 slice fresh pineapple
1 glass of orange juice
1 glass of water

Lunch
Fish
1 potato or rice
Salad
1 glass of water

Snack
A small pot of low fat yogurt

Dinner
Fish any style
Vegetables
Salad
1 glass of water

As you can see these particular eating and drinking plans do not include any eating or drinking habits that are:

1.   Too fattening.
2.   Too sugary.
3.   Too salty.
4.   Too heavy and starchy.
5.   Too fizzy or unnatural.

This type of eating and drinking plan should be implemented seven days a week for really FAST weight loss. If you stick to a good diet plan seven days a week, you are more likely going to lose weight much faster.

If you are somebody who finds it difficult to stay away from those eating habits that you know make you put on weight, then what you could do is have one day in the week that you could eat and drink some of your favorites, but the most important thing is for you to get back on track on your good diet plan the very next day.

If you have chicken, or red meat, then it is very important that you go for the leanest cuts, that is chicken without the skin on, and red meat that has less fat around it.

PLEASE NOTE: These diet plans that I have outlined are just guidelines for you to follow so that you can lose weight FAST, but they do not have to be followed religiously.

For example, instead of having fish for lunch you could have chicken or steak instead. Instead of having eggs for breakfast with a slice of bread, you could have instead sardines or salmon slices with some beans and salad. Instead of having a potato you could have a small portion of rice. Your portion sizes of salad, vegetables, rice or oatmeal should not be too big, but in small portions.

Water

If you really want to break down body fat FAST, then it is very important that you incorporate water into your daily plan for greater success. Most people who are trying to lose weight do not drink enough water.

That is why they tend to have a problem trying to lose weight FAST. Weight gain is generally as a result of high levels of FAT that have accumulated inside our bodies over a period of perhaps days, weeks, months, and even years of our lives, eating foods and snacks that are really high in fat content, and consuming heavy amounts of food and drinks each day.

This slowly piles up in our body system. And the best way to break down the accumulation of body fat is to drink lots of water each day which is going to help us to flush out and remove the accumulation of fat from our bodies.

This is also going to be VERY POWERFUL when we combine it with regular physical exercise and a good diet. Whenever I have had to lose weight in the past, before I do fat burning exercise I have at least two cups of herbal tea.

Afterwards, I would have a large glass of fresh drinking water. This helps me to break down high levels of body fat by 100 percent whilst I am doing a workout session.

Drinking in this way over a consistent period of time seven days a week is a sure way to help you to lose weight, feel healthier, cleanse and purify your body system, giving you very good skin, and making you look younger.

Drinking water is one of the key, fundamental, and most powerful ways for you to lose weight FAST. Aim to drink at least 2 pints (just over a liter) of water each day.

THE RIGHT TYPE OF TRAINING PROGRAM FOR FASTER WEIGHT LOSS

Dieting alone can make you lose weight but, if you want to get rid of stubborn body fat FAST around the areas of your body that you are not happy with, then regular physical exercise should be implemented as your strategy and plan for greater success.

Somebody who implements regular exercise with a good diet plan is going to lose weight much faster than somebody who implements only a good diet. Physical exercise with regards to losing weight really means the constant movement and the shaking up of the body system for long periods of time – let's say for example between twenty and ninety minutes.

This creates internal heat within the body system, which enables you to break down high levels of body FAT around the areas of your body that you are not happy with. In order to do this by exercising, there are certain exercises that you would need to do on a regular basis that are going to GUARANTEE that you cannot fail in this particular area of your life that really matters.
Over the course of twenty years I have discovered the most effective exercises for losing weight FAST. These are as follows:

1. Jogging.
2. Fast walking (power walking).
3. Circuit training.
4. The step machine.
5. Boxing.
6. Kick boxing.
7. Skipping (with a rope).

8.   Sprint training.
9.   Interval training (high intensity type of exercises).
10.   Resistance training, e.g. bodyweight or weight bearing exercises.
11.   The stair master.
12.   Abdominal exercises (fast movements).

For the best results

For the best results it is very important that you do a combination of some of those very effective exercises that I have just mentioned between three and six days a week without fail. In order to burn body fat much more effectively you would need to incorporate the following SUCCESS strategies.

1.   Endurance training (long distance).
2.   High intensity type exercises.
3.   Resistance training using your own body weight or doing weight bearing exercises.

People who combine these three success strategies into their weekly training program are going to lose weight much faster than those people who do not.

Endurance training

Endurance training means the ability to maintain the effort whilst exercising to lose weight for periods of thirty to ninety minutes in order for your fat burning workouts to be really effective. In terms of endurance training I am talking about doing the following:

1.   Fast walking (power walking).
2.   Jogging.

3. The stair master.
4. The exercise bike.
5. The step machine.

These exercises must be performed at quite a slow pace if your fitness levels are low. If your fitness levels are at a medium level then these exercises will have to be performed at a moderate pace. If your fitness level is really high then you would need to perform this type of exercise at a moderate to fairly fast pace.

High intensity exercises

High intensity types of exercise are by far the most effective way for YOU to lose weight FAST. In terms of high intensity exercise, I am talking about doing exercises that are going to be taking you out of your comfort zone and that would be making you work at 60,70,80,90 and 100 percent effort at times, requiring a lot of focus, and a lot of determination.

Somebody who does this is going to lose weight three to four times faster than somebody who does not. By high intensity types of exercise, I am talking about the following:

1. Sprint training.
2. Skipping (with a rope).
3. Kick boxing circuit training (for weight loss).
4. Boxing circuit.
5. Circuit training.
6. Spinning classes.

People sometimes say, "Oh, I have been exercising and dieting for quite some time but I have not been losing weight." I can GUARANTEE that they have not been APPLYING this type of high intensity exercise that I have just mentioned above into their weekly plan to lose weight FAST. High intensity exercises should be applied not less than twice a week.

Sprint training

Sprint training is a fantastic way to burn body fat FAST and the best way to do so is to do the following:

a.   50 yards or 50 meters
b.   100 yards or 100 meters
c.   200 yards or 200 meters

If you are not used to sprinting in any way, I would suggest that you first go for three 50 yard (or 50 meter) sprints twice a week, doing them at 70 percent effort if it is your first time. When you finish doing each sprint, walk back to the start position.

It is very important to make sure that you warm up first by jogging for fifteen to twenty minutes, loosening out all of your joints for five minutes and then stretching.

When your fitness levels are starting to get better, increase the 50 yard sprints to six or seven times doing the first three sprints at 70 percent, the fourth at 80 percent and then the remaining sprints at 100 percent effort. When you start to become accustomed to this type of training, you could progress into doing 100 yard sprints.

CAUTION: If you are not used to jogging, then sprint training is not advisable. To progress into sprints, you must have been jogging for several weeks.

This type of training is going to make you really tired, but at the same time it makes you SWEAT and BURN a lot of CALORIES. This would take your fitness to a really high level within three to four weeks if you performed those drills on two or three days a week.

In order to get the best results, you need to put a lot of power into the movements, which means you need to have strong arms (upper body strength) and also strong legs (lower body strength). This means you are going to have to strengthen and tone your whole body on no fewer than three days a week in order for you to get the best benefits and results.

Skipping

Skipping with a rope is by far one of the most effective ways to lose weight FAST. It is definitely not a favorite exercise for most people who need to do so, but I am going to say that it really WORKS especially for those people who are prepared to do what is NECESSARY in order for them to get the results that they want to achieve. An example of a good skipping program is as follows:

1. Skip for two minutes.
2. Rest for one minute.

Perform these very effective exercises five times round, which is going to be a total time of fifteen minutes. Before skipping, do a fast walk or a jog for 15 minutes.

Resistance training

Resistance training is really weight training, or body toning. It's important to include it in your training program if you really want to lose weight FAST. Most people, who need to do so, do not know about the importance of incorporating weight training into their plan to get the results that they want.

If you do this you lose weight much faster than somebody who does not. The benefits of resistance training if you include at least three and do them three times a week are as follows:

1.   More STRENGTH
2.   More POWER
3.   A more SHAPELY and TONED BODY
4.   And FASTER WEIGHT LOSS.

In order to lose weight FAST by doing resistance training, it is very important that the movements are really done in a fast way. I am talking about combining different exercises, let's say for example:

1.   Jogging on the spot: one minute
2.   Bent over rows: one minute
3.   Jogging, combined with sprinting on the spot: one minute
4.   Squats: one minute.

This should be done with really fast movements using weights that are medium to light, performing a continuous circuit of three– so twelve minutes in total – and then moving on to the next very effective set of exercises which are as follows:

1.   Jogging, moving or on the spot: one minute
2.   Press ups: one minute
3.   Sprinting on the spot: one minute
4.   Power cleans: one minute
5.   Sit ups: one minute

Perform this particular circuit three times, which is going to be a total time of fifteen minutes.

NOTE: The total FAT burning, body toning, and strength workout is going to take twenty-seven minutes. For exercise illustrations and techniques, please go to section 6.

Technique

For burning body fat effectively the right use of technique is important. Most people who exercise to lose weight do not apply the right type of techniques whilst they are exercising, which means they could be burning body fat by only 10, 20, and not more than 50 percent each time that they do a workout session.

Doing so without the use of proper form and technique makes losing weight extremely difficult. If you want to get rid of stubborn body fat FAST, then you need to APPLY the right techniques, body positioning, and movements.

This will help you to BURN body fat by 100 percent, making your workout sessions very productive and efficient. The right use of techniques can be developed over a consistent period of time, until it becomes a part of your life.

THE AMOUNT OF FAT THAT YOU CAN BURN BY DOING EXERCISE

By doing physical exercises regularly you can BURN the following amounts of calories:

Infinite calories
1000 calories
900 calories
800 calories
700 calories
600 calories
500 calories
400 calories
300 calories

The MORE calories BURNED whilst you are doing physical exercise, the more BODY FAT you are going to get rid of. For you to lose weight, it is very important that you BURN much more than you consume.

For example, diet plan number four is not more than 500 calories so, if you are implementing that particular diet plan daily, each time that you exercise you should be looking to BURN much more than 500 calories.

What I generally do in order to lose weight FAST is aim to burn up to 1000 to infinite calories by doing the most effective FAT burning exercises, six days a week.

This I do by putting in two to three hours of exercise each day. For example thirty minutes early in the morning, and ninety minutes in the evening. I also try to stick to a 500 calorie diet each day.

There are times that I do not always follow that particular guideline, which means that I sometimes have a day or two when I eat up to 700 and even more than 1000 calories, but the good news is that I am still going to lose weight FAST, because of the 1000 or infinite calories that I would have burned by doing the most effective FAT burning exercises.

MINDSET

If your mind is not set on making losing weight a total MUST in your life then, unfortunately, all the best information and knowledge in the whole world on how to lose weight will come to nothing. You have to be ready to IMPLEMENT and APPLY what you know. Mindset includes the following mind strategies:

a.	Taking action.
b.	Using the power of focus.
c.	Positive words and thinking.
d.	Mental strength.
e.	Determination.
f.	The power of visualization.
g.	Being consistent and committed.
h.	Discipline.
i.	Patience.
j.	Rest.
k.	The achievement of your weight loss goals.

What I have just mentioned are the ELEVEN GOLDEN RULES of how the mind should operate and function in order for you to get the results that you want. In order to succeed, all of those points must be in PERFECT HARMONY.

For example if you don't take action then you are not going to get the results that you want. If you were to take action but you were not really committed, disciplined and focused on achieving the results that you want then you are not going to succeed.

Taking action

There is nothing more powerful than taking action on what you know you need to do. Doing so is the blueprint and the solution to your weight gain problems and issues and your desire to be who you really want to be deep down as regards your shape and health.

Most people in the western world who need to lose weight fail to take action because for most people it is an extremely hard road to follow, to eat and drink healthily and to control one's food portions consistently.

It is also very difficult for most people to exercise regularly. Deep down we want to eat and drink whatever we want without being so organized (disciplined) with eating and drinking habits and also to stay in our comfort zone by not applying regular exercise.

This eventually causes much frustration, unhappiness and lack of fulfillment in a person's life who knows they need to lose weight but they lack the motivation to do so. I am going to call that situation being in a WEIGHT GAIN PRISON because they want to be "FREE" from weight gain, but the road ahead seems too hard and difficult (sticking to a daily diet and exercising regularly). This ultimately leads to a person becoming "TRAPPED" in a weight gain prison by their own choices. This comes with a host of negatives, such as the following:

1. I feel unhappy about my shape.
2. I hate myself.
3. I feel so unhealthy.
4. My clothes do not fit anymore.
5. I used to be so slim and fit before.
6. I feel tired most of the time.
7. My sex life is being affected.
8. I feel bloated and heavy most of the time.

9. I am suffering from low self-esteem and have no confidence.

If you are experiencing any of those negatives due to weight gain, by taking immediate action straight away by exercising regularly and being on a good diet plan, you are going to be moving away from any of those negatives, and by being consistent you are eventually going to experience the positives, which are the following:

1. I really feel happy about my shape.
2. I like myself.
3. I feel so healthy.
4. My clothes fit me well.
5. I am slim and fit.
6. I feel energized most of the time.
7. My sex life is better.
8. I feel light and active inside most of the time.
9. My self-esteem and confidence have improved greatly.

All of these very positive emotions and feelings are there for you if you take ACTION straight away and do so over a consistent period of time. It could be days, weeks, months, and a year or even in some cases years, depending on one's weight loss goals. The most important thing is to go in the right direction toward who you must really become deep down.

Remember the old saying:

"ACTIONS SPEAK LOUDER THAN WORDS"

So it is time to take ACTION until you become the person that deep down you really want to be, as regards your body and health.

Using the power of focus

If you want to SUCCEED then you must use the power of focus. You must use the power of focus when you are about to exercise and also whilst you are exercising to lose weight.

Doing so with 100 percent commitment and focus on your training is eventually going to give you 100 percent benefit and results. The power of focus is about using the MIND–BODY CONNECTION as regards losing WEIGHT around the areas of your body that are making you unhappy.

This means FOCUSING your entire mind whilst you are training to really BURN body FAT by 100 percent. Most people who exercise to lose weight do not use the POWER of CONCENTRATED EFFORT and FOCUS on what they are doing.

So most people find it extremely HARD to lose weight and get the results that they are really looking for because whilst they are exercising they allow their minds to wander and to be sidetracked by the following:

1. Work.
2. Money.
3. Relationships.
4. Family.
5. Other thoughts, things and issues.
6. Speaking on the phone.
7. Watching the television.

If you want to get 100 percent results from your workouts, then you need to LEARN how to switch your mind OFF from any distractions, and really FOCUS 100 percent on your workout.

The human mind is extremely POWERFUL if it really focuses on a task. Over the course of many years, I have sometimes asked my clients while they have been training, "What are you thinking of right now?" They generally mention other things besides losing weight.

This means that they are not FOCUSING 100 percent on losing weight, and that they are not going to get the results that they really want. Under the POWER OF FOCUS, it is very important to be single-minded and really FOCUSED on the task at hand, whether you are exercising for twenty minutes, sixty minutes or ninety minutes.

Positive words and thinking

It is very important to use the POWER of POSITIVE words and thinking when wanting to exercise, or whilst exercising to lose weight, saying for example:

1. I CAN LOSE WEIGHT.
2. I WILL LOSE WEIGHT.
3. I WILL SUCCEED
4. I CAN BECOME THE PERSON THAT I WANT TO BE.
5. I AM A CHAMPION.
6. I MUST DO IT
7. I AM VERY DETERMINED.
8. I MUST WIN.
9. I ACHIEVE MY MOST IMPORTANT GOALS.

If you want to succeed, these are the kinds of words that you must imprint in your mind's eye each day, and get rid of any negative words and thinking in your mind that says "YOU CAN'T".

So many people who I have come across over the years stop themselves from losing weight because they have reasons why they can't lose weight which I am going to call the NEGATIVES. The negatives are the following:

1. I do not think that I could ever lose weight.
2. I cannot lose weight, no matter how hard I try.
3. Being overweight, it is just a part of who I am. It tends to run in my family.
4. I don't think that I could ever be slim.
5. I am just too old to lose weight.
6. I cannot lose weight because I have got a thyroid problem.
7. I cannot lose weight because I am going through the menopause.
8. I cannot lose weight because I am on medication.
9. I don't think that I could ever break this weight loss barrier.

Those are some of the most common objections, the reasons why so many people cannot lose weight. In most cases if somebody cannot lose weight, it could have something to do with their daily diet e.g. they could be eating too much carbohydrate in the form of bread, rice, pasta, dumplings or potatoes or eating and drinking things that are sabotaging their success.

It could also mean not sticking to a strict seven day diet by breaking it occasionally. For somebody who has got the diet part right, they may not be exercising regularly or applying the right type of training program to lose weight FAST.

There is always a solution to a weight gain problem. But it is about believing that it is POSSIBLE and that YOU CAN LOSE

WEIGHT. Do you have any negative objections as to why you cannot lose weight?

If you do, I am going to ask you to set them aside, and I would like you to say to yourself, or out loud that:

IT IS POSSIBLE

Say it again

IT IS POSSIBLE

And again

IT IS POSSIBLE

And it is really going to be POSSIBLE if you believe that YOU CAN and you IMPLEMENT the SUCCESSFUL weight loss STRATEGIES that I have been talking about in this book.

Mental strength

In order to succeed in this particular area of your life that really matters, you are going to need a lot of mental strength and focus.

Programming your mind to have that positive self-talk most of the time is eventually going to give you the ability to acquire great mental strength and focus on what you need to do in order to WIN.

Mental strength is also having the ability to keep on going forward when you don't feel like doing any exercise or sticking to your healthy eating and drinking plan. Mental strength can be developed by the following:

1.   Employing a personal trainer.
2.   My audio version of this book.
3.   Your friends, family or partner.
4.   Having the right motivated training partner.
5.   Enrolling in a gym.

MENTAL STRENGTH DURING PHYSICAL EXERCISE

You are going to need a lot of mental strength and focus whilst you are exercising to lose weight in order for you not to quit and to ensure that you complete your workout sessions. Great mental strength is required for the following:

1.   To help you get started.
2.   For you to stick to the plan.
3.   For you to complete what you have started.
4.   For you to be really consistent.
5.   For you to burn much more from your workout session.

Using GREAT MENTAL STRENGTH whilst training is going to help you to BURN more CALORIES and ACHIEVE– as opposed to somebody without mental strength.

Determination

One very powerful quality and trait that you must possess if you want to lose weight FAST is determination. Somebody who is extremely determined to lose weight fast can be very powerful.

There are many people who say that they want to lose weight but many do not do so because they lack the determination to succeed. Determination in my definition is having a strong, burning desire to succeed in this particular area of our lives that really matters.

For somebody who is determined to lose weight, they are generally prepared to do what is NECESSARY in order to succeed which means if they need to exercise for one hour or more, five or six days a week, they are going to do so without making excuses as to why they can't.

They are generally prepared to implement a healthy eating and drinking plan by getting rid of certain eating and drinking habits that could be stopping them from ACHIEVING. If they are taken off track by occasionally not implementing regular exercises and eating and drinking in the right way, they would generally get back on track on the road to shape and health SUCCESS.

A person who is very determined NEVER GIVES UP on their shape and health GOALS. When somebody says "I can't lose weight" determination comes into play by saying "I CAN LOSE WEIGHT. When somebody needs to lose weight by exercising but they just don't feel like it, determination comes into play by saying "I MUST DO IT."

Determination is the driving force which is going to lead to your SUCCESS as regards your weight loss goals. It is also going to help you to overcome the following:

1.   Obesity.
2.   Inactivity.
3.   Negative words such as "I CAN'T LOSE WEIGHT".
4.   Procrastination (putting off doing something that needs to be done).
5.   Stubborn body fat.
6.   Laziness.
7.   Bad eating and drinking habits.

The lack of determination on the other hand is going to lead to the non-achievement of your weight loss goals (FAILURE) which means you are not going to lose weight or reach your ultimate weight loss goal – or break out of your WEIGHT GAIN PRISON.

That means you could remain as you are or even become worse as time goes by. To be determined, think about what you LOVE as regards your shape, health and wellbeing, and also what you dislike and HATE as regards your shape, health and wellbeing.

If you were to do this type of thinking on a regular basis that would hopefully give you more determination to SUCCEED.

The power of visualization

The more you keep on thinking positively about losing weight, the more chances you have of SUCCEEDING. It is very important to visualize and see your body the way that you would like it to be on a constant basis, and keep on saying to yourself that you are going to be that person that you really want to be deep down.

Visualize the daily healthy eating and drinking plan that you would need to have, and follow it in your mind's eye each day, Monday right through to Sunday for four weeks. Also visualize yourself doing the most productive workout sessions that you would need to do in order to SUCCEED.

Think about and visualize how you are going to feel after doing a good workout session. This could be that apart from feeling tired you are now feeling these positives:

1. I now feel great.
2. I feel so healthy.
3. I really feel energized.

4. I now feel less stressed and more motivated.
5. I feel really happy.
6. I am so glad that I talked myself into doing exercise.

Be consistent and committed

Once you take ACTION by exercising and eating and drinking healthily, you must then decide to be consistent with applying what you know is going to be beneficial for you. Being committed to this way of life does not just mean that you are committed because you are going on holiday in a few weeks' time so you need to lose weight FAST and then you go back to your old habits of no physical exercise and bad eating and drinking habits. It should be about being consistent with healthy eating and drinking on a daily basis and regular physical exercise. Be committed and say to yourself that:

REGULAR EXERCISE AND HEALTHY EATING AND DRINKING IS FOR LIFE

Say it again

REGULAR EXERCISE AND HEALTHY EATING AND DRINKING IS FOR LIFE

And again

REGULAR EXERCISE AND HEALTHY EATING AND DRINKING IS FOR LIFE

"And the reason is that there are going to be massive benefits for me if I do so."

Discipline

You must set rules and regulations as to what you can eat and what you must not eat, how many days you are going to exercise, and your rest days, and then STICK to them.

If you do this, you will eventually become that person that deep down you really want to be. Discipline is going to be one of the hardest and greatest challenges that you will face in this respect, but the good news is that this powerful force that is called discipline can be learned and mastered if you are determined to make it a part of your life.

Being disciplined is eventually going to give you personal fulfillment, joy and happiness in this particular area of your life that really matters.

Patience

Most people who need to lose weight FAST become impatient whilst they are trying to do so –they want to achieve quick results and success overnight. They fail to take into consideration that losing weight is an inch-by-inch process which means it really takes time and effort.

For example in section 1, I mentioned that the general guideline for somebody to lose weight is to lose 2 pounds every week so, in a twenty-eight day period, 8 pounds, which is 3.6 kilos. Some people who want to lose weight start on a Monday and check the scales on the Tuesday, and then the Wednesday, and Thursday, becoming obsessive about whether they have lost weight.

When they discover that they are not getting the results they wanted to achieve before the end of the week, they start to become de motivated, stressed, frustrated and unhappy, saying to themselves that this losing weight business does not work. The main issue here is that this person is FAILING to be PATIENT and stick to the guidelines and rules which are to aim to experience weight loss by the end of the week and to keep on being persistent until they reach their goals.

GOOD ADVICE: If you want to lose weight FAST you must learn how to be patient, and to develop persistence and determination.

Rest

If you are exercising regularly to lose weight, it is very important that you get enough rest in the form of sleep each day, which means that you generally need eight hours of sleep.

This is crucial. Somebody who is well rested, who gets their full eight hours of sleep that is so needed for their mind and body, is going to be able to put more power and energy into their workouts.

Thus they are going be able to burn and lose weight much FASTER compared to somebody who does not sleep enough and is tired throughout the day.

So it is very important that you get the amount of sleep that you need each day, so that you can recharge your batteries and feel really energized and motivated in order for you to be able to put in the time and energy into your FAT burning workouts.

The achievement of your weight loss goals

This is when you become really happy; this is the time that you feel a sense of joy, personal fulfillment and happiness, in this important area of your life.

This is the time that you have IMPLEMENTED all of the most necessary weight loss strategies to give you the results that you have wanted. You achieved your weight loss goals because you took ACTION, you achieved your weight loss goals because you NEVER GAVE UP and also you achieved your weight loss goals because you had the desire and the determination to SUCCEED.

You also achieved your weight loss goals because you realized and understood that the non-achievement of it was not an option or choice that you were ready to settle for but the achievement of your weight loss goals was something that you had to LIVE WITH and BE.

GREAT TIPS FOR MORE WEIGHT LOSS

With regard to exercising to lose weight, it is very important to do this on an empty stomach. So if you are going to exercise in the morning try not to eat anything beforehand so that you can burn body fat by 100 percent instead of burning the food first instead of your body fat.

If you exercise in the afternoon or evening then it is important to eat something really light like fruit three hours before. After your FAT burning workouts, wait for an hour before you eat, so that the fat burning heat that you created can be harnessed and developed fully all over your body system for up to an hour. Food will reduce the fat burning effect process.

It is also very important before you are about to exercise to have one or two cups of hot water with lemon and honey or herbal tea and then have a large glass of water. All these strategies are definitely going to give you the edge over the great majority of people who need to lose weight FAST but find it hard to do so because they lack the understanding of the best success strategies to apply in order to get the fast results that they really would love to achieve.

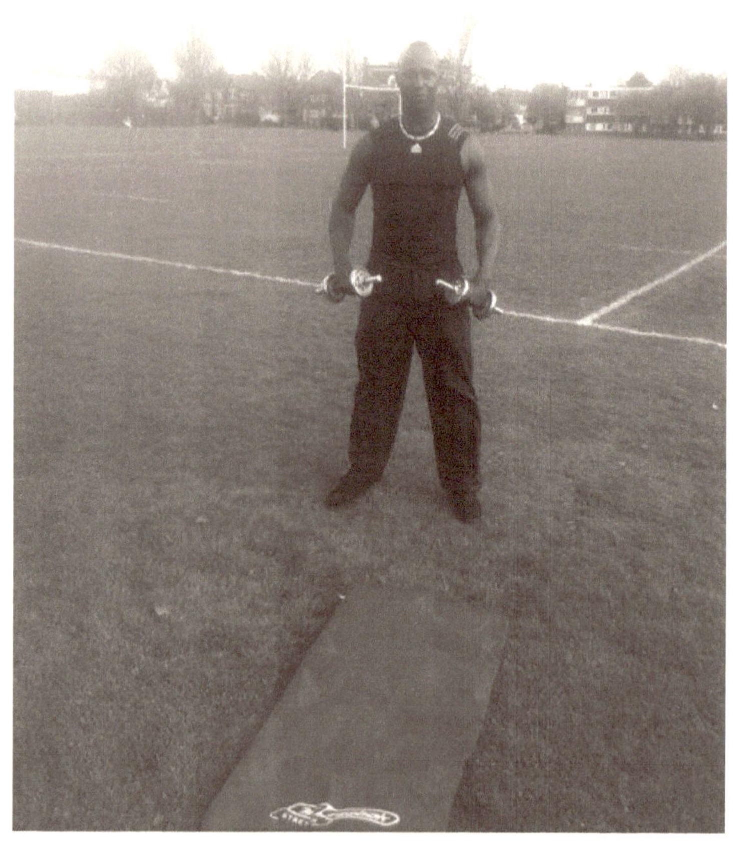

DUMBBELL SIDE RAISES

It is very important to keep your back straight. Look slightly up. Your feet should be wider apart than shoulder width. Have a set of dumbbells or two bottles of water if you haven't got any.

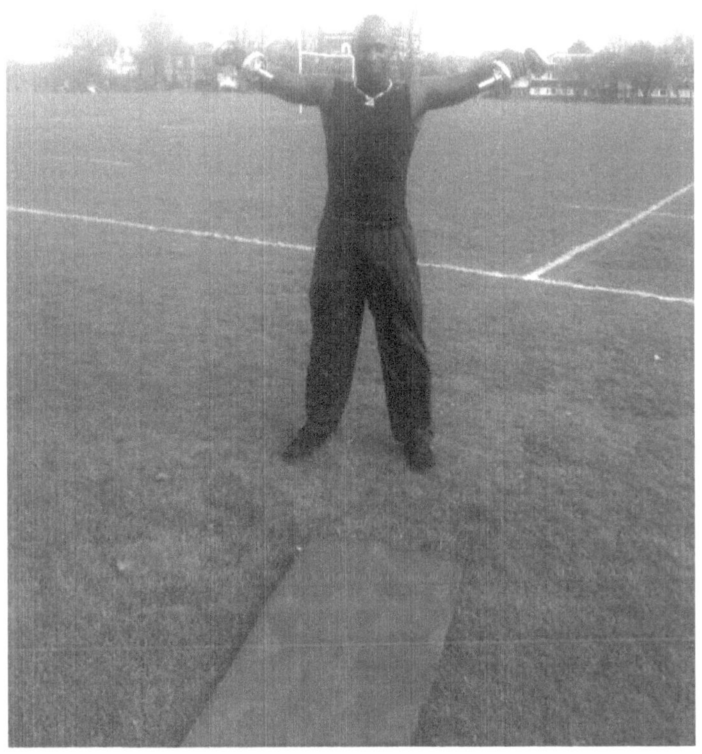

Now raise the dumbbells above the shoulders in line with the top of your head. Your arms should be slightly bent when performing this particular exercise. You need to raise the resistance weights in a fast movement for really FAST weight loss.

These exercises work the side of the shoulder muscles. And secondary muscle groups worked are the arms.

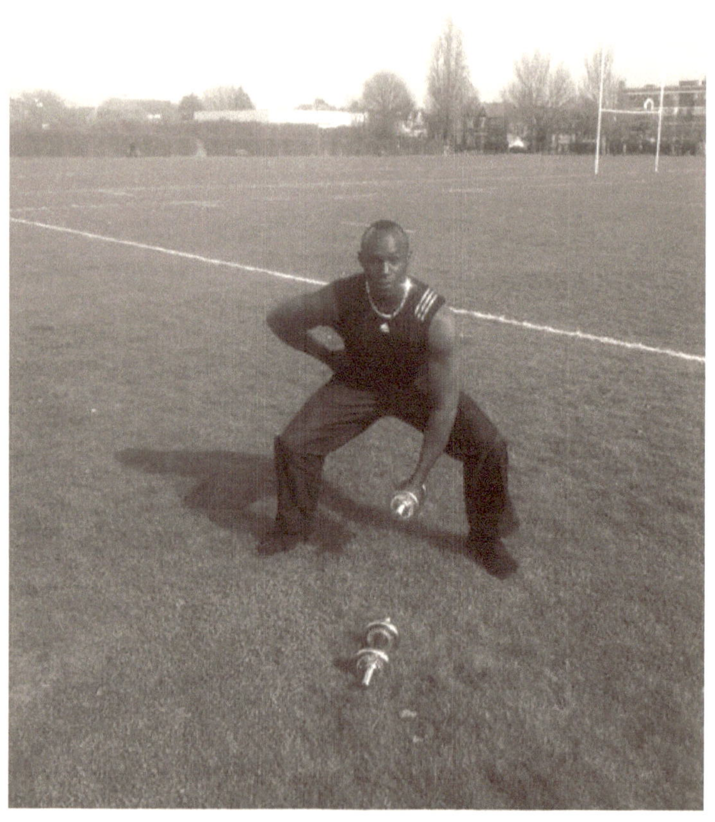

ONE ARM DUMBBELL SIDE POWER RAISES

For this particular great exercise, you use only one dumbbell. Your other arm that is free touches your hip. Stand up straight. Your stance should be wider than your shoulders. Then go down in a squatting position, making sure that your back is straight and your head is in a forward position.

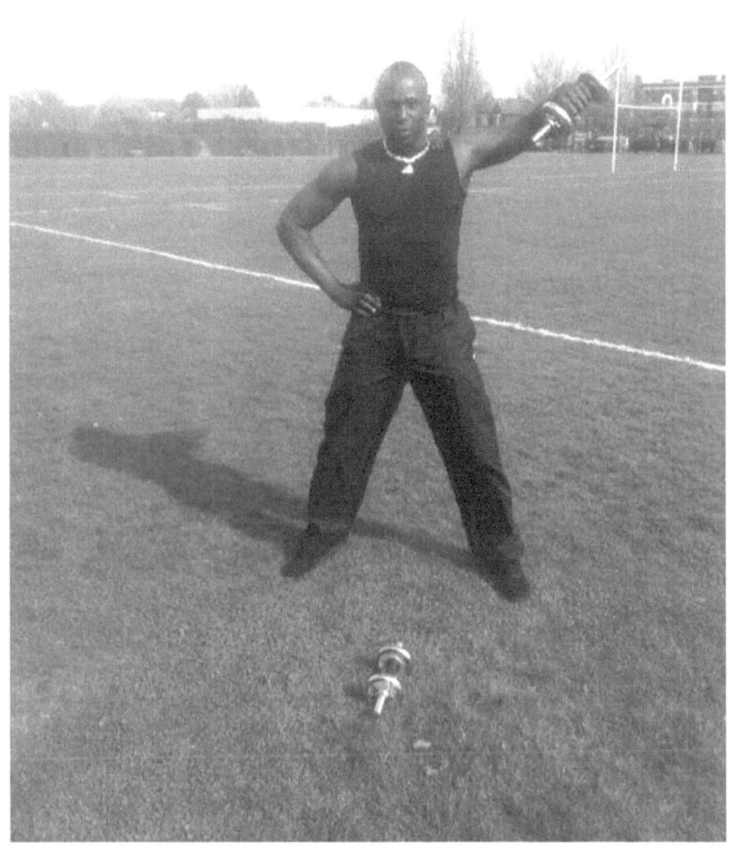

Then use your thighs to push your body up, raising the dumbbell at the same time, above your shoulder and level with the top of your head. It is also very important when you raise your body up to go onto your toes. This exercise works the thighs, the side of the shoulder, your arm and the calves.

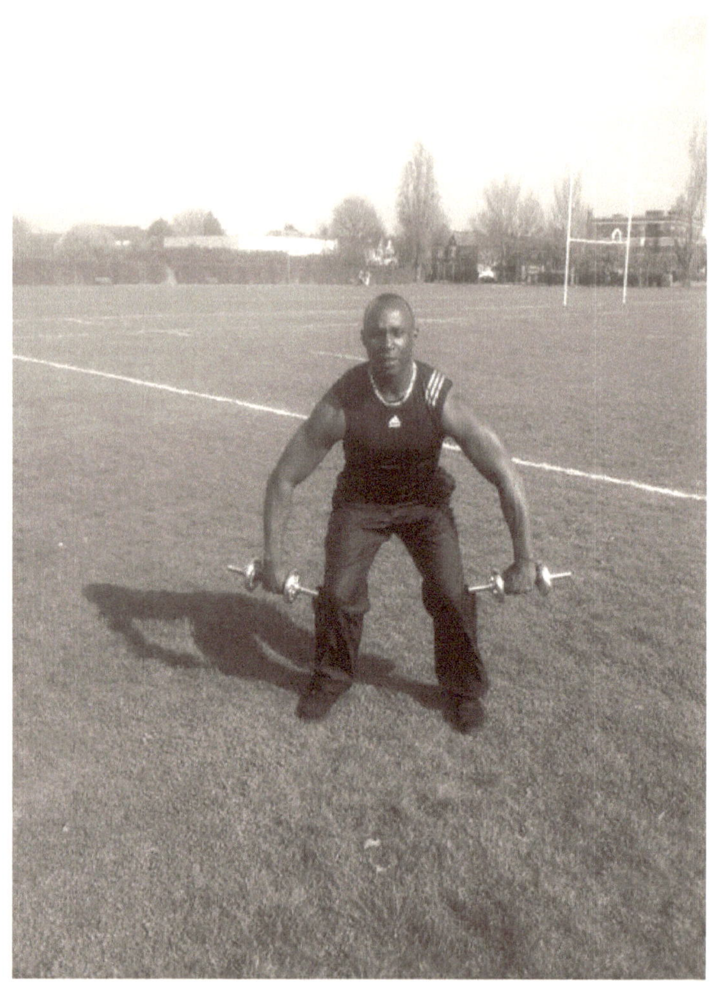

DUMBBELL POWER CLEAN

This is a fantastic exercise for increasing your metabolic rate and for you to burn body fat really effectively around your stomach area. Start by standing straight. Your feet should be shoulder width apart with your head held high. Your arms with the dumbbells should be to the sides of your body. Now bend down into a squatting position, bending your knees, with your back straight and your head looking forward.

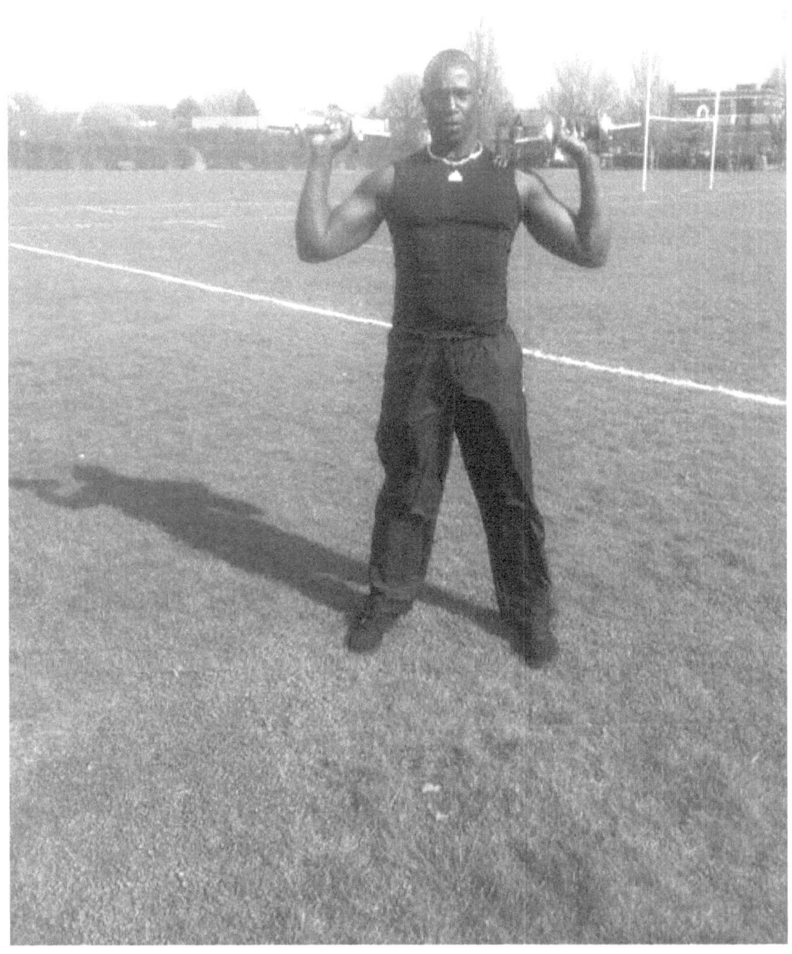

Then raise the dumbbells up to shoulder height and back down into the start position with your arms to your sides. Perform this particular exercise for 30 seconds.

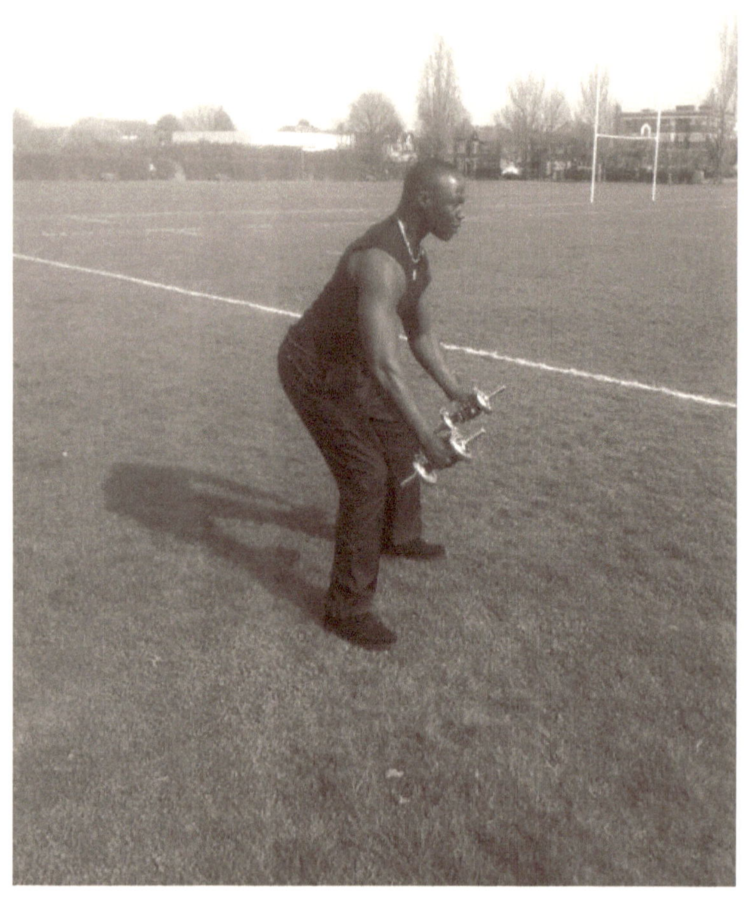

THE DUMBBELL BENT OVERROWS

This is one of the best exercises for burning body fat around the stomach area has well as other parts of your body. It also works your middle back muscles, your biceps and your forearms. Hold a set of dumbbells. Bend your knees, keep your back straight, extend your arms and look forward.

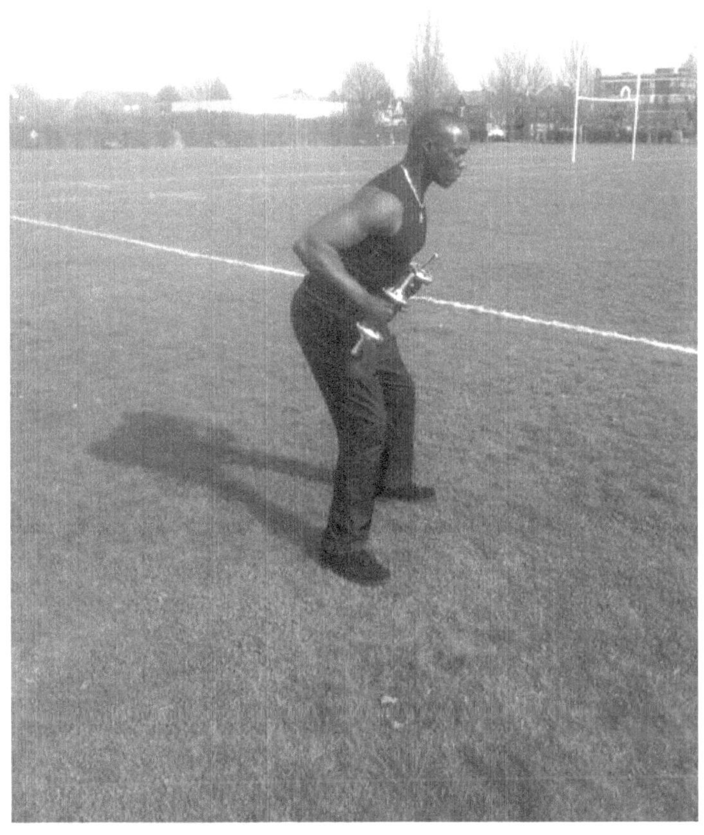

Now raise the dumbbells up below the chest and squeeze the back muscles. And again back down to the start position. These movements should be done really FAST, putting great power and speed into the movements.

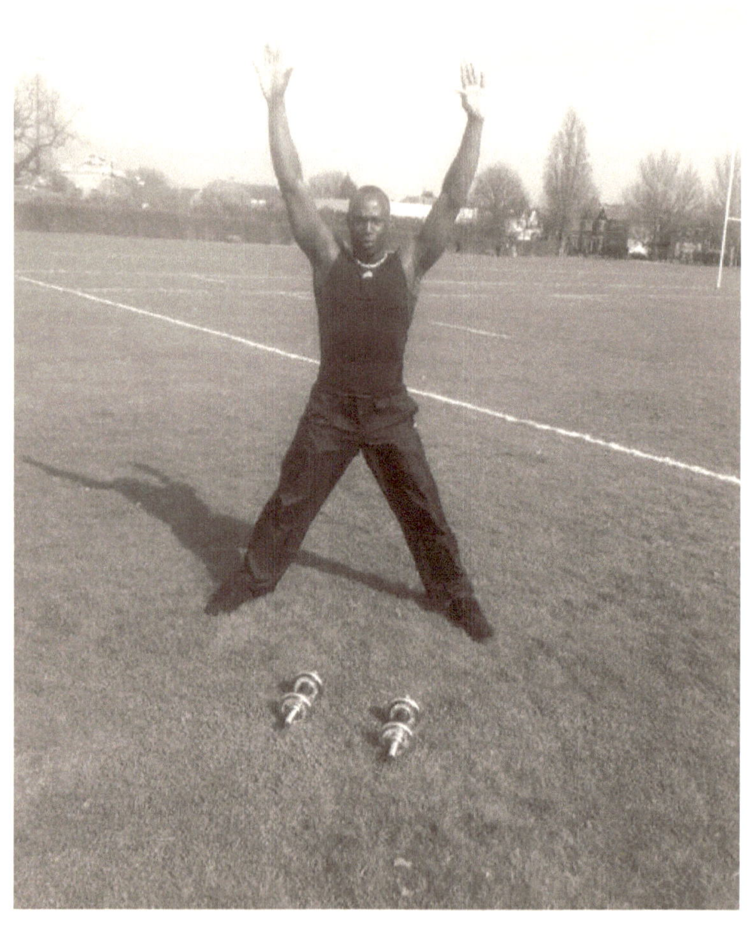

SQUATS

This exercise works your respiratory system, your heart and lungs, increasing your fitness levels and also works your bum and thighs. It is also a fantastic FAT burning exercise when performed in a fast way.

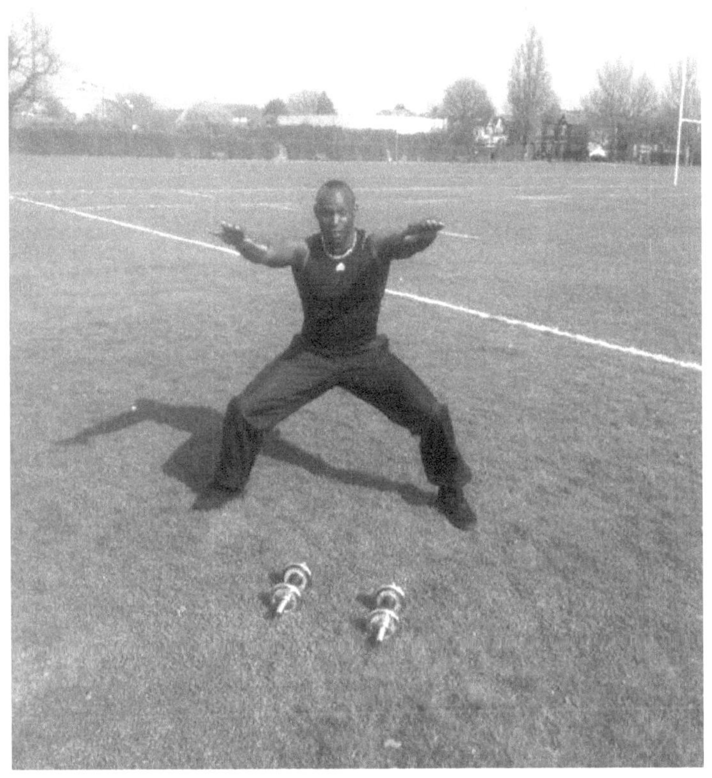

Go down and up, ensuring that your legs are positioned wider apart than shoulder width, and keep your back straight. You can perform these exercises with your arms fully extended overhead or in front of your chest. For added resistance, you could use a set of dumbbells held level with the top of your shoulders or to the sides of your body.

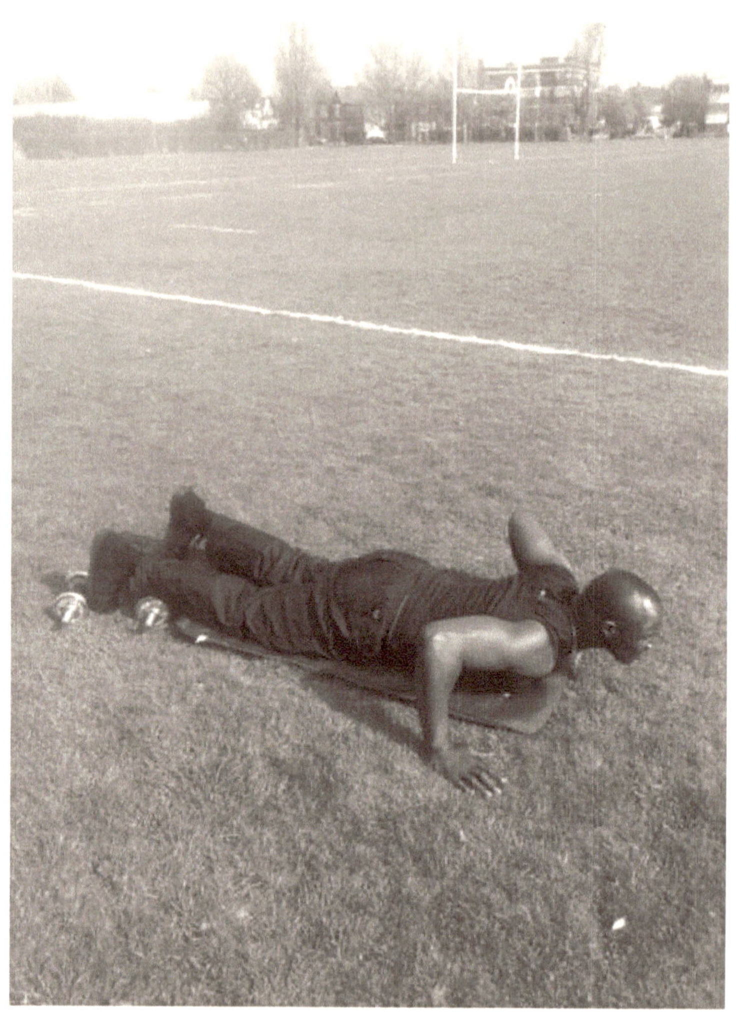

PRESS-UPS

This is a good exercise for increasing your upper body strength and also your fitness levels, when done in a fast way. The muscles worked are your chest and the triceps muscles which are at the back of your upper arms.

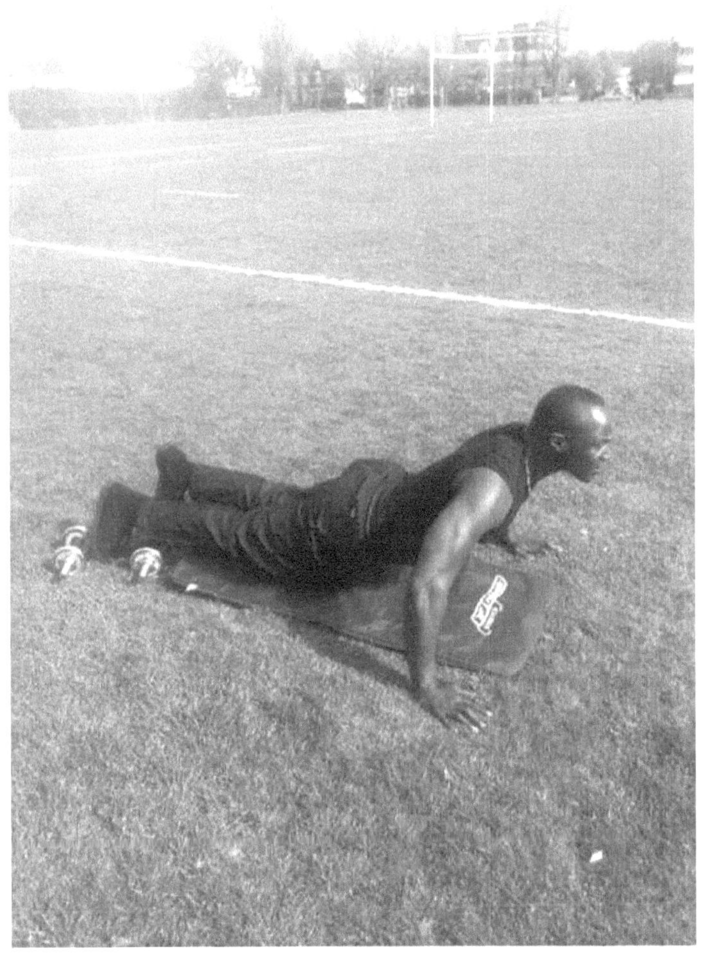

Keep your back straight, lie down onto your chest, position your fingers and your arms in line with your shoulders. They should be 10 inches away. Now push your body up using your arms, ensuring that your knees are off the ground. If you lack upper body strength, then an easier version is to do this particular exercise with your knees touching the ground at all times.

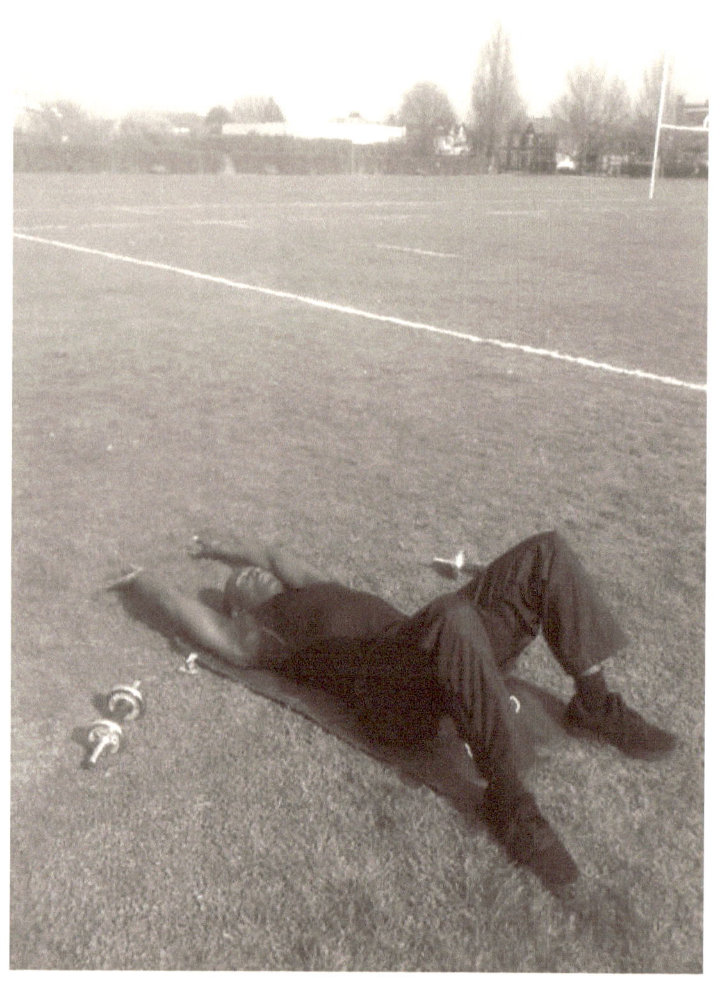

SIT-UPS

This exercise is for toning and burning body fat around the stomach area especially if it is done in a fast way instead of slowly. Start by lying down on your back. Stretch your arms over your head and bring your knees up, with your feet touching the ground.

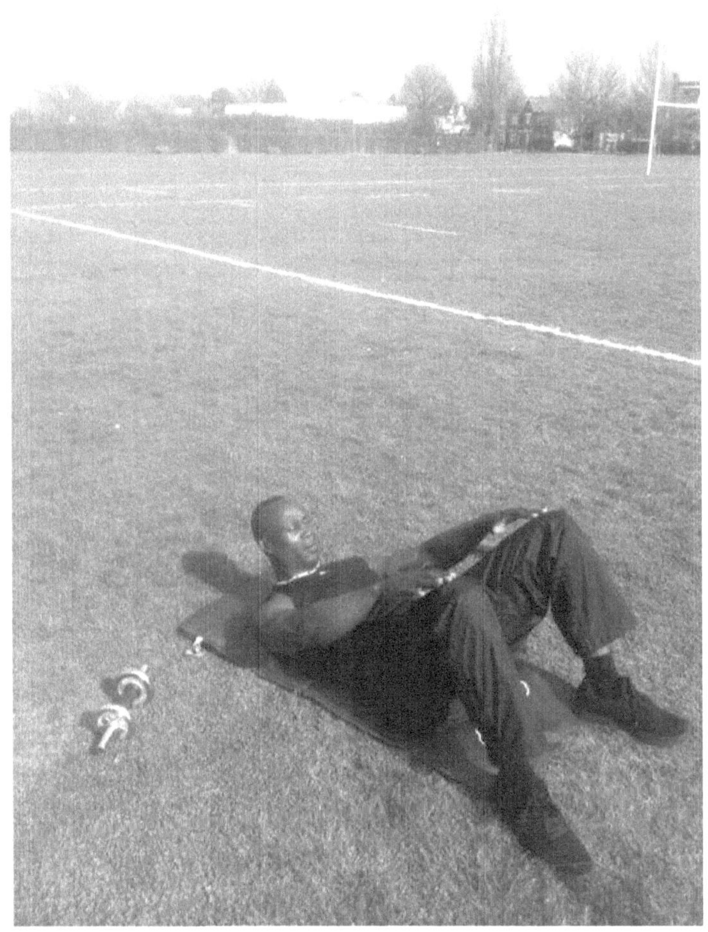

Raise your body up; your fingers should touch your knees at the top. And go back down into the start position. Perform those movements really FAST for more weight loss and increased fitness levels.

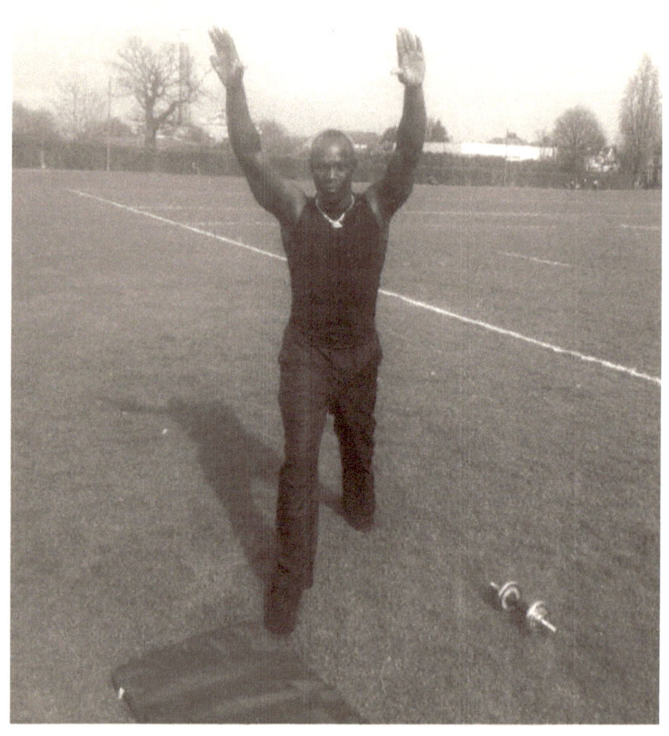

STANDING ONE-SIDED KNEE RAISES

This is a very good exercise because it helps you to get a good stretch when the back foot is brought up to stomach level with the knee bent and your fingers brought down to touch the knee.

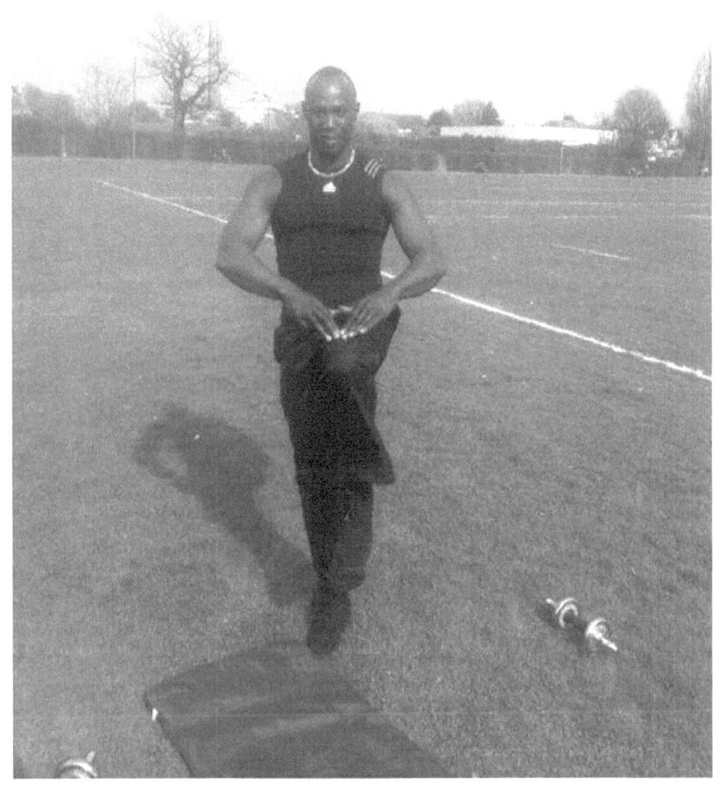

This becomes a terrific and powerful fat burning exercise when done in a fast way. Start off with your right foot, do it for thirty seconds and then change to your left foot and do it again for thirty seconds.

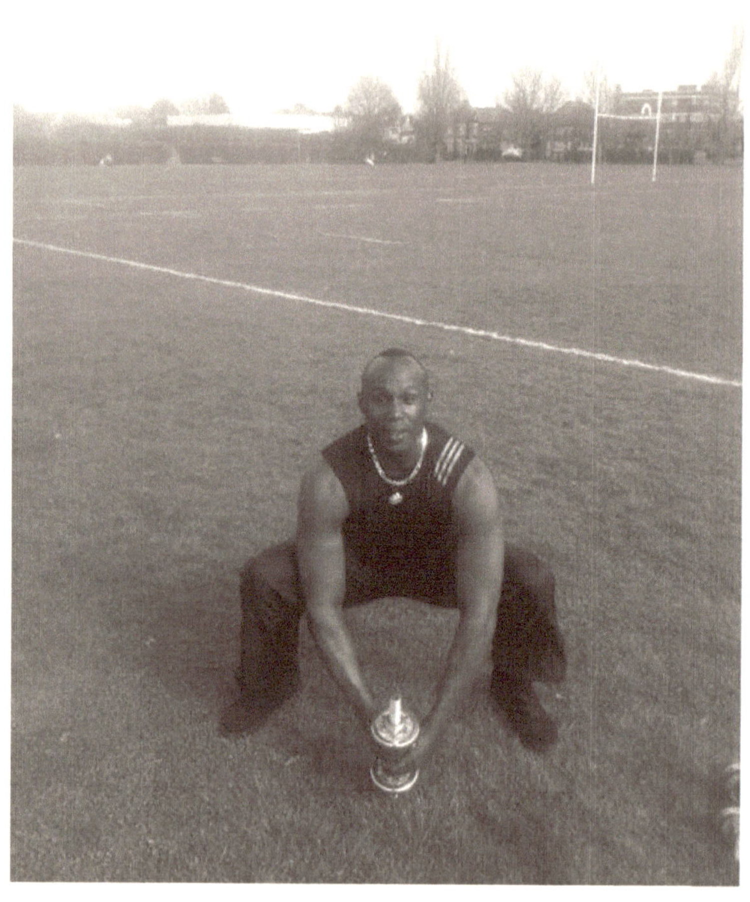

ONE ARM DUMBBELL OVER HEAD RAISES

This exercise strengthens your arms, your thighs, bum and calf muscles and also your lower back. Start by holding one dumbbell, your chest and your head held high. Your back should be straight, and your feet should be wider apart than shoulder width. Go down into a squatting position, bending your knees.

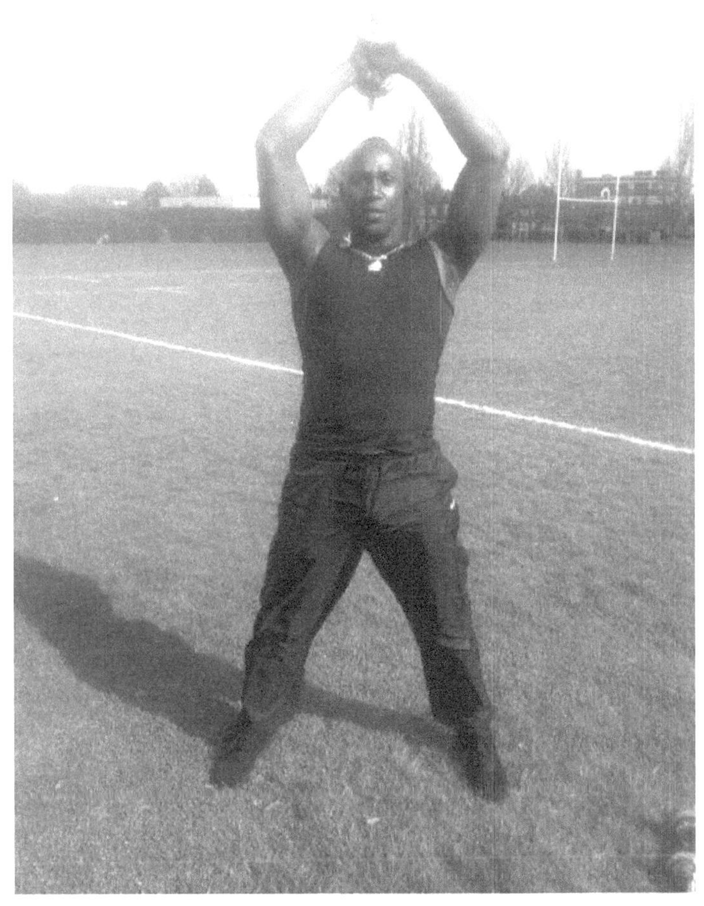

Raise the weight right up over your head and go up onto your toes. And back down into the squat position and right up once again. Perform this particular exercise for 30 seconds.

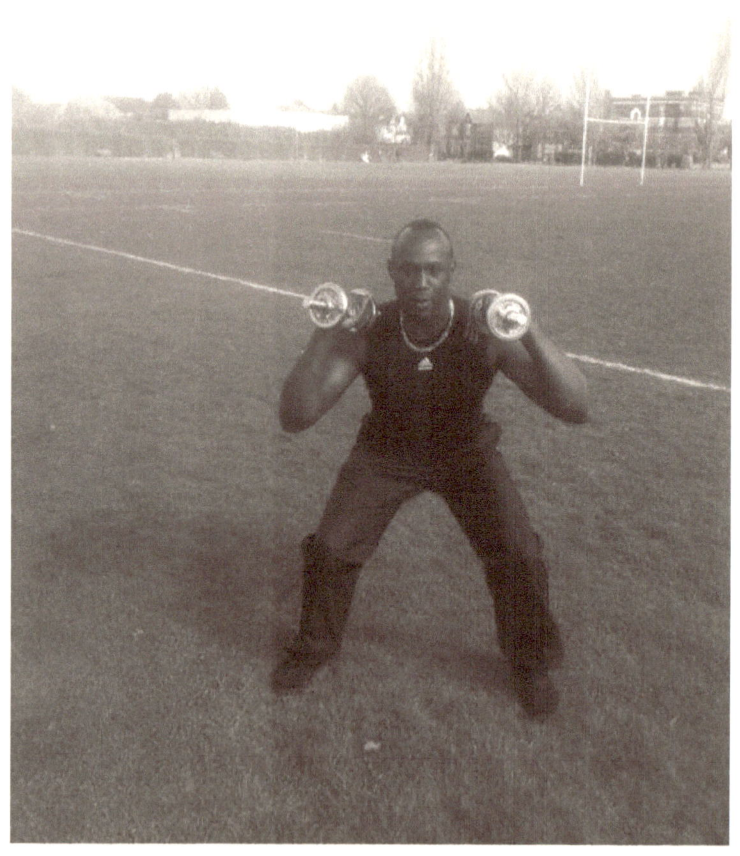

PUSH PRESSES

This is a fantastic exercise for working the thighs, shoulders, arms and the calf muscles. You start by standing straight, holding resistance dumbbells in your hands in line with your shoulders. Your feet should be positioned wider apart than shoulder width. Go down into a squatting position.

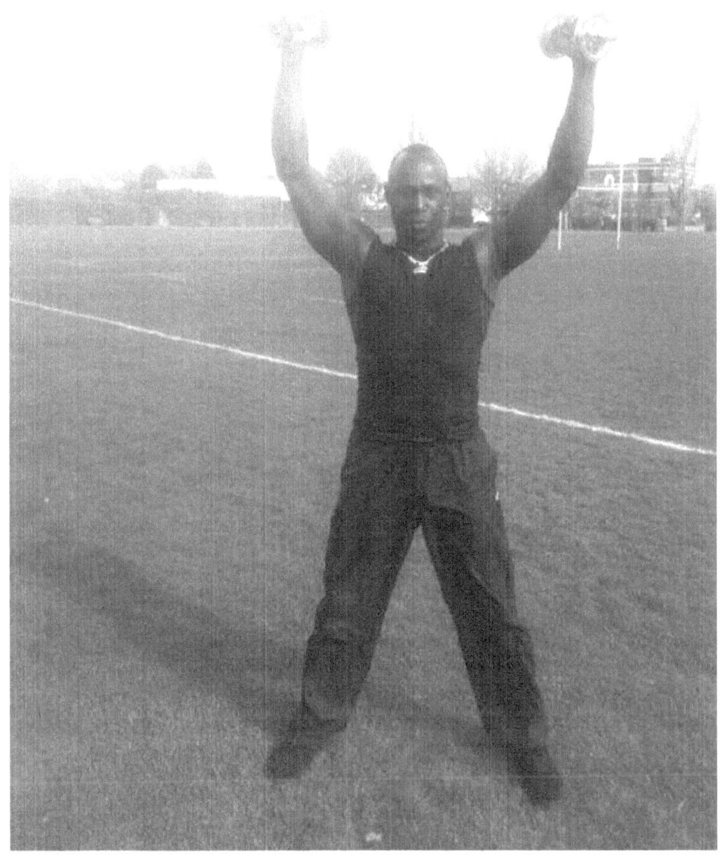

And then push up using your thighs and your calf muscles to extend your upper body, extending your arms high above your head. Do not fully extend your arms, but ensure that they are slightly bent at the elbows.

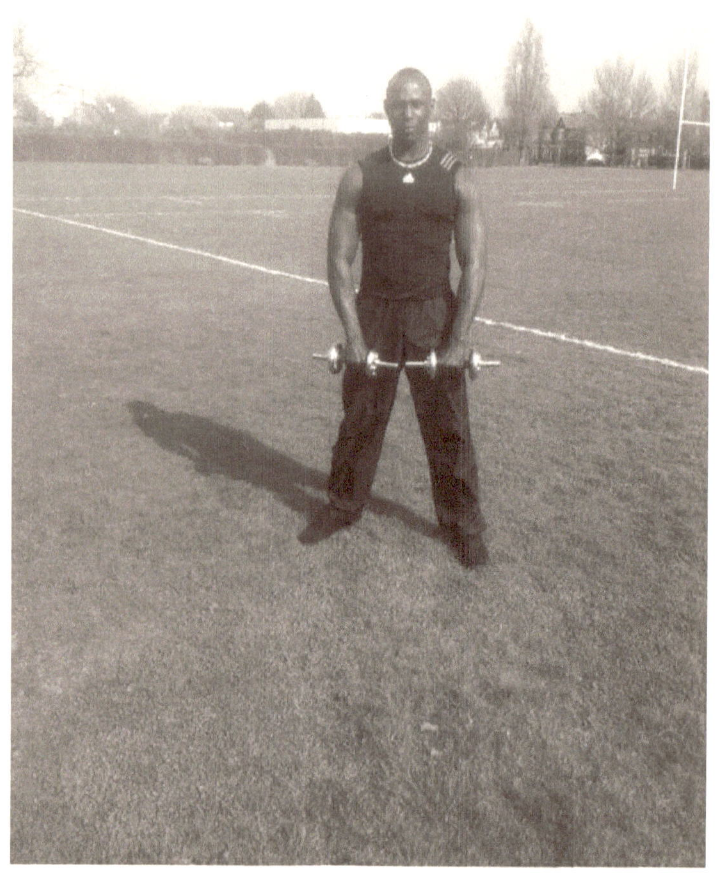

UPRIGHT ROWS

This is a very good exercise for working the arms; especially the area between the neck and the shoulders called the trapezium muscles. Keep your arms down with a slight bend.

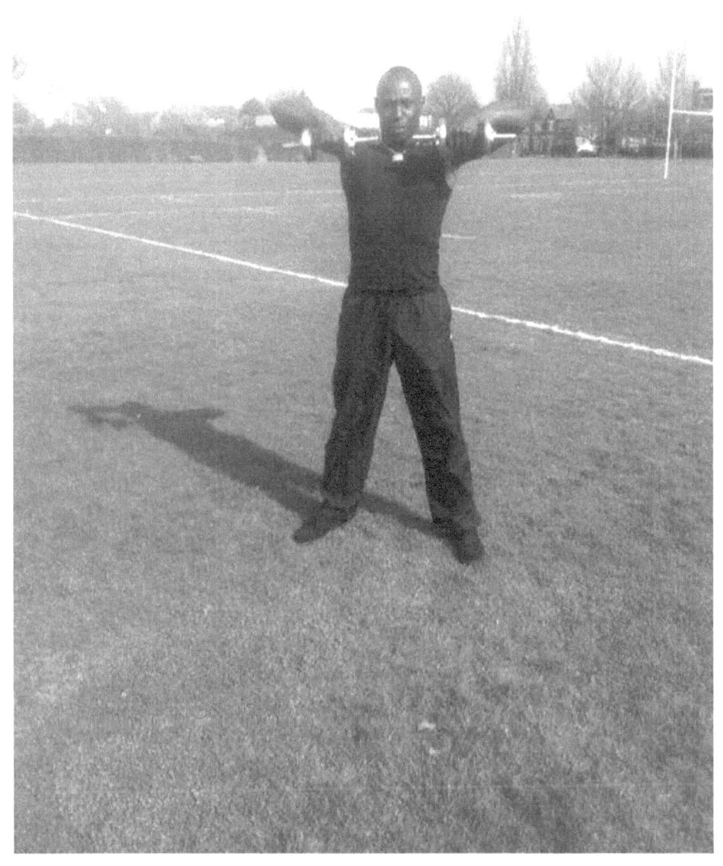

Now raise the weights up slightly below your chin. From the top, lower them once more under control to the start position. Now raise them up and down, up and down using the mind–body connection.

I hope you enjoyed this book!
The author may be reached via email or website.
Email: mitchsoul@rocketmail.com
Website: www.mitchfitness.com
Tel : 07875508603